C000302370

THE FOOT CARE BOOK

An A-Z of fitter feet

By Judith Kemp SRCh
City and Hackney Health Authority, London

Edited by Lee Bennett
Age Concern England

About the Author

Judith Kemp has been working as a state registered chiropodist in the National Health Service for the past ten years. During this period she has also done research into the need for and provision of foot care for an MSc degree, which was published as Problems Afoot. *She also works in the research field with the Age Concern Institute of Gerontology.*

© 1988 Age Concern England
Bernard Sunley House
60 Pitcairn Road
Mitcham
Surrey CR4 311

ISBN 0-86242-066-0

Designed by Eugenie Dodd

Illustrations by Robin Dodd

Production by Joyce O'Shaughnessy

Typeset from disc by Parchment (Oxford) Ltd

Printed by Ebenezer Baylis and Son Ltd The Trinity Press, Worcester

Contents

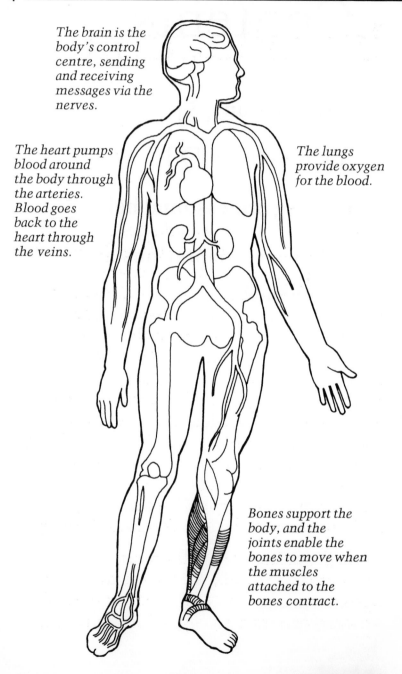

The brain is the body's control centre, sending and receiving messages via the nerves.

The heart pumps blood around the body through the arteries. Blood goes back to the heart through the veins.

The lungs provide oxygen for the blood.

Bones support the body, and the joints enable the bones to move when the muscles attached to the bones contract.

Introduction

Three out of every four adults have foot problems, though most people are born with normal feet. Some of these problems are inherited, some are caused by a lifetime of wearing ill-fitting shoes, others result from illnesses which develop in middle and old age. Because the systems and structures of the body (as shown opposite) are so inter-related, any illness which affects them may also affect your feet. This book explains about foot conditions, everyday care and how to choose shoes for comfort. The guidelines are presented so that you can take responsibility for improving your comfort and understand when to get specialist help.

Though our feet may be the most downtrodden parts of our bodies, they are the basis for an active and independent lifestyle for everyone from the age of one onwards.

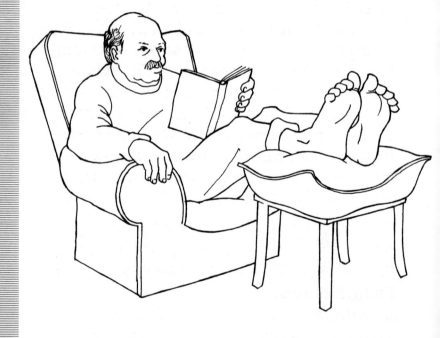

An $\boxed{\textbf{A-Z}}$ of feet

This section of the book contains information about foot conditions with guidelines on self-care, when to seek professional treatment and what to do in an emergency – when, for example, you may have sprained your foot. In addition the common illnesses of middle and old age are discussed for people who may be affected by arthritis, diabetes or poor circulation. Exercises to maintain healthy ankles and feet as well as guidance about nail care have also been included.

The drawing of the foot overleaf can be referred to when a particular problem may have altered the way your toes lie or your foot functions.

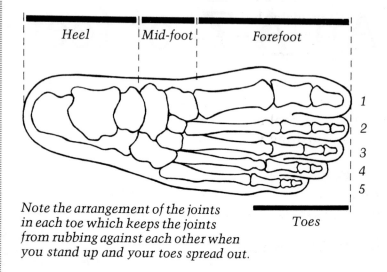

Note the arrangement of the joints in each toe which keeps the joints from rubbing against each other when you stand up and your toes spread out.

A Aching feet

This condition is all too common and is usually caused by standing still for a long time in unsuitable shoes or by having to walk long distances when shopping or doing housework.

Home remedies Choosing properly fitting shoes is the essential long-term remedy. Wearing support hosiery can also help.

For instant relief, lie down or sit with your feet raised higher than your hips for 15 minutes, as shown on page 6. When lying down, rest your feet against the wall or on the arm of a sofa or pillow. Raising the feet above hip level allows gravity to help drain away fluid which accumulates in the feet and ankles. In walking, the calf muscles help to move this fluid upwards, but when you are standing or sitting still the muscles are not working.

Contrast footbaths may also be beneficial. Plunge the feet into a bowl of warm water for 1 minute, then into a cool bowl for 15 seconds. Repeat 3 to 4 times, finishing with a warm one.

Professional treatment The GP can advise about any underlying deformity or disease, and a chiropodist can recommend footwear.

■ **Ankles,** *see page 48.*

■ **Arthritis**

The cause of this condition is not clear, but the result is a painful joint with restricted movement as the surfaces of bones become rough and distorted. In severe cases the bones may fuse together which relieves the pain but prevents any movement.

Osteoarthritis

This is a thinning and wearing down or roughening of the cartilage that covers the ends of the bones at the joints. The main symptons are painful, creaky joints. The bigger weight-bearing ones such as the knees and hips are usually affected before the fingers and toes.

Home remedies Before treating yourself, get a professional diagnosis, as you may have gout, rheumatoid arthritis or other conditions which require investigation and medical treatment. Unless you are told *not* to, try the following methods of self-treatment:

Painful joints need rest to allow the inflammation to subside and then, gentle exercise. For toes, hold either side of the affected joint and, very gently pull your hands apart to move it. By repeating this about 6 times daily, there should be a small increase in the range of movement and a lessening of pain. Massaging the skin with an emollient cream like Simple Ointment BP is another way of moving the joints passively. Try to exercise them by wiggling your toes in a warm bath and rotating your ankles.

Gentle heat also helps ease pain, but be very careful not to burn your skin, especially if your circulation is not good. A hot water bottle should be covered in a fabric cover or wrapped in a towel to help prevent skin damage.

Professional treatment A GP may prescribe pain killers. A physiotherapist will try to improve movement of affected joints and may use heat to ease the pain and electrical stimulation to strengthen muscles. He/she may also advise on gadgets to help with putting on hosiery and shoes. A chiropodist may also suggest manipulation, will advise on footwear, and may prescribe (and make) an insole to help foot function and relieve pain.

Surgery may be suggested for severely painful osteoarthritis to remove the affected joint.

Rheumatoid arthritis

This affects the muscles and skin as well as the joints and is more common among women between the ages of 25 and 55. It first affects the small joints in the hands and feet. There are acute phases – which may last from a few weeks to several months – interspersed with periods of some respite. However, once damaged, the joints will remain so.

Its affect on the toes pulls them up and backwards and away from the ground. The fatty pad which usually lies beneath the joints joining the toes to the foot is pulled forward, and the joints are thus separated from the ground only by a thin layer of fibrous tissue and skin. Under such pressure and deprived of natural cushioning, the skin develops callouses. If left untreated, the skin will eventually split, or an ulcer may form and affect the tendons in the foot.

Home remedies, see professional treatment.

Professional treatment Drug therapy is used to control the inflammation and is balanced with treatment to keep joints mobile and as strong as possible. In acute phases, joints must be rested, and lightweight splints may be prescribed to immobilise them. Warmth is useful in reducing pain, but care must be taken to avoid burns or overheating. To keep the muscles from wasting, try tensing and relaxing them without moving the joints; and repeat this several times an hour. After an acute phase you should try to move the affected joint and do exercises to retain mobility, but get a chiropodist or physiotherapist to advise.

A chiropodist will explain what you can do to relieve pain and avoid ulcers. He/she will treat hard skin and corns and attempt to deflect pressure from painful areas, usually with removable padding or insoles. The typical deformity of rheumatoid feet means that extra depth is required in shoes to accommodate both the foot and a padded insole. A physiotherapist may also be involved in treatment, providing splints and muscle building exercises, especially during an acute phase.

Surgery is often performed on rheumatoid feet, when the joints at the base of the toes are removed and the fatty pad is pulled back into position, so that you no longer walk 'on the bones'. Although this is a major operation, the relief gained can be considerable.

■ Athlete's foot

This skin infection appears as reddish, shiny patches, with scaly edges which may sting or be very itchy, though the centre of the patch may look quite normal. Between the toes where the skin is moist, the affected area will look white, soggy and peeling.

Home remedies Apply surgical spirit between the toes, twice a day, immediately after washing the feet. If this doesn't cure the problem, try one of the anti-fungal creams or lotions available at a pharmacy.

To affected areas on the top or sole of the foot, apply anti-fungal cream, and always continue the treatment for at least 4 weeks after the symptoms have disappeared to clear the cause of the condition. Wear clean hosiery daily, and disinfect shoes with an anti-fungal talc or spray.

Professional treatment A doctor or chiropodist may take a small scraping from the skin surface for examination in the laboratory and will suggest treatment as described for home remedies.

B Blister

This is a sac of fluid which occurs close to the surface of the skin, and results from friction, burns, infection, skin diseases, or insect bites. The fluid is usually clear but if the blister occurs deep in the skin, some blood may leak into the fluid, turning it pink or red. If the blister bursts, there is a risk of infection, and it may become painful as the raw surface comes in contact with the air.

Home remedies Try not to burst a blister – just cover it with a clean dry dressing. If it is burst, clean the area and apply antiseptic ointment to a clean non-stick dressing.

If it is really necessary to burst the blister, use a sterile needle, and make two punctures, at opposite sides. Use cotton wool to apply pressure and then put on a dressing.

To avoid getting a blister from new shoes, do not

wear them for long periods initially. Correctly fitted shoes should not rub, but they may be harder than old ones. Lumpy seams can be hammered (protecting the surfaces of the shoe with a cloth) to soften them.

Professional treatment Multiple blisters, or ones with no obvious cause, should be shown to the doctor for diagnosis and treatment.

■ Bunion

This deformity of the big toe causes it to lie at an angle instead of straight ahead. The second toe may lie over the big one or be buckled under it, and the rest of the toes may be pushed out of alignment. Other conditions such as a bursa, corns and ulcers may occur with a bunion.

Home remedies There is no effective home remedy; but you can prevent the big toe being pushed further across by choosing shoes of the correct shape – that is, with a straight inside edge (see page 61).

Professional treatment The only effective treatment is surgery. There are numerous variations of the operation, the choice depending on the exact nature of the deformity and the surgeon. Most chiropodists do not carry out surgery on bunions, although they may do so in the future. They will advise about the soft tissue problems connected with bunions and may provide protective padding (see page 71).

■ Bursitis

This is inflammation of a bursa, a sac filled with fluid found in various parts of the body. In the foot, a bursa commonly forms over a bunion to protect the joint from excess pressure. If the bursa is irritated it becomes swollen, hot, red and painful. In very severe cases the fluid may be forced through to the surface and be discharged.

Home remedies Remove pressure and friction on the bursa by resting the foot and being careful about footwear. To relieve swelling, raise the affected foot to hip level when sitting. A cold compress will soothe and cool the area – use water or a mild astringent like witch hazel or aluminium acetate, which evaporate easily. If this treatment works and the skin is unbroken with no discharge present, try to prevent bursitis recurring by working out the original cause. If there is a break in the skin, keep the wound clean and covered and get professonal help.

Professional treatment The doctor may prescribe antibiotics and dressings to prevent infection or may refer you to a chiropodist or a district nurse for similar treatment. In very extreme cases, surgery may be necessary.

C Chilblains

These are small, itchy, red areas of skin, caused by exposure to damp, cold and draughts. If broken, they weep a clear fluid.

Home remedies Don't scratch chilblains. An antiseptic dressing is only necessary if a chilblain has broken, but a dry dressing may reduce itching.

To prevent chilblains, wear trousers, long socks (woollen or thermal), tights to keep legs warm, especially if you have to stand at a bus stop in cold, damp weather. Boots which cover the ankle may also help. Housebound people should avoid sitting in draughts and should wrap a blanket around the legs and feet if the room is cold.

Professional treatment A chiropodist or GP may suggest an ointment or liquid to prevent itching and promote healing.

■ **Circulation,** *see page 33.*

■ **Corn**

This area of thick skin has a hard core which is pushed into the surrounding flesh and causes pain. It is cone shaped, with the pointed end imbedded in the skin and the wide area at the surface. As corns are caused by pressure, try to work out whether badly fitting shoes or slippers may be restricting the movement of toes. If corns are less painful in summer, shoes may well be causing them.

Hard corns are the most common and generally form on the soles of the feet, on the tops and tips of toes, on bunions or on bony parts of the foot. Some corns have small blood vessels in them which appear on the surface as a small black dot.

These vascular corns bleed when cut and are sometimes confused with a verruca.

Soft corns form between the toes, are whitish and rubbery in texture because the skin gets waterlogged with sweat and from being washed.

Home remedies Do *not* cut corns unless you want to give your doctor or chiropodist extra work. Instead, use a pumice or hard-skin stone or chiropody sponge regularly to remove the thickened skin a little at a time. Be wary of corn plasters, lotions and solvents that contain acid which burns the hard skin – and the soft surrounding skin – as a burn or cut can become infected.

To relieve pressure between the toes, insert a foam or felt wedge or a ring which can be removed at night. A tubular foam cover worn on one toe has a similar function. Felt rings may also help, so long as they do not contain an acid medication. When using any of these cushions, be sure that they are not making your shoe tight and causing pressure elsewhere. Avoid using lambs wool as it has a tendency to shrink when damp or wet; and when wrapped around a toe, can shrink and cut off circulation – causing severe swelling, pain and even gangrene.

Professional treatment A chiropodist will pare away the hard skin and remove the core with a scalpel, which does not usually cause bleeding or pain. A chiropodist may also use an acid to remove the core, or soften the area, even though self-treatment with acids is not advised. The corn may also be burned away or frozen (particularly for a vascular or neuro-vascular one). A local anaesthetic, given by injection, may be needed for these treatments.

Once the corn has been removed, padding may be applied to relieve the area from pressure. Obviously, pads will wear thin and become less effective, but must remain in place. For corns on the soles of the feet, insoles may be the answer. To ease the pressure on toes – or to make room for a prominent joint like a hammer toe – a balloon patch may be inserted or the upper of the shoe stretched.

It is not usual for a doctor or surgeon to treat corns, although a GP may do so where no chiropodist is available. If corn plasters or solvents are recommended by the GP, take care to follow the instructions on the packet and remove the plaster at any sign of trouble.

■ Curly toes

With this condition, the toes no longer lie straight and flat on the ground. The tips may point downwards, or may be rotated so that the nails no longer appear on the top of the foot. If the condition is longstanding, the joint surfaces may be permanently deformed. Other terms for curly toes used by a chiropodist or doctor are claw, mallet, hammer and retracted.

Home remedies If there is still some movement in the toes, it may be possible to strengthen the muscles by exercise. Try stretching the toes out straight, with the foot off the ground. Gentle manipulation may also ease pain and increase the movement of the joint.

Professional treatment A GP may refer you for chiropody or surgery. A chiropodist will provide padding or occasionally surgery. A surgeon may attempt to straighten the deformity in a variety of ways: the joint may be removed and the bones joined, giving a rigid toe; or a false joint may be created by inserting a plastic replacement or allowing a fibrous joint to form.

|D| Dermatitis

This is a general term for a variety of skin problems which can affect any part of the body. Contact dermatitis is caused by an irritating substance which makes a red, slightly swollen and itchy area on the skin. For example, some people react to biological washing powders, while others are affected by the zinc oxide in sticking plasters or the dyes used in shoe making (easily recognised when the affected area conforms to the shape of the shoe upper). Sometimes the lanolin, fragrance or colour used in skin creams is the cause.

Home remedies A mild antiseptic lotion will cool the affected areas, until you have identified what is causing the problem. If the dye used to colour the leather in shoes is an irritant, the manufacturer may be able to identify the chemical involved and help you to avoid making another unsuitable purchase.

Professional treatment If you cannot identify the cause of the irritation, ask the GP for a referral to the dermatologist to have 'patch tests' for sensitivity.

Eczema

The cause of this problem is unknown, but it can be associated with asthma and is most commonly found in adults who had attacks in childhood. It frequently occurs on the legs, and can be very uncomfortable and unsightly, though not infectious.

Home remedies Use good quality unscented soap for washing, and pat the skin dry rather than rubbing it. Keeping cool can reduce irritation, but unbearable itching should be rubbed, not scratched. Clothing should be rinsed extra carefully, and it is best to avoid wool next to the skin. Try to avoid getting agitated, as stress can make eczema worse.

Professional treatment Skin creams or lotions may be prescribed, containing ingredients such as coal tar or steroids. Use these strictly as prescribed — more may not be beneficial.

Pomphlyx

This shows as a very itchy, burning patch of small blisters, commonly found on the soles of the feet and the palms of the hands. There is no home remedy, and you should consult your GP.

■ Diabetes

If you have diabetes, you lack insulin to move sugar from the bloodstream to the cells where it is needed for growth and repair. If the level of sugar in the bloodstream rises too high, it begins to appear in the urine.

The effects of diabetes are an increased risk of hardening of the arteries and of a blockage or thrombosis (see page 37). The eyes, kidneys, legs and feet are frequently affected by impaired circulation; and the reduced blood flow may also result in a loss of sensation in the ankles and feet and feeling pins and needles (see Insensitive feet, page 31).

Because of the reduced sense of pain or pressure, you may not notice cuts or bruises on your feet, burns, scalds or frostbite. As the skin may also become undernourished, it is less resistant to damage or infection. Because of poor circulation and impaired healing, diabetics are more prone to infections, which can become severe if not treated promptly (see page 30).

Home remedies Being careful about your diet (to keep the blood sugar level normal) is the first essential aspect of home treatment. A daily foot inspection is the other. Because of reduced sensitivity in the feet, check for cuts, blisters, corns and areas of skin which have been reddened or indented by seams in hosiery or shoes. At the same time, check footwear for embedded nails in the soles and the inside of the shoe for rough or crumpled insoles or cracked uppers.

Before washing your feet, test the temperature with a thermometer which should not read more than 40c 105f. When toenails need cutting – provided you can see properly – follow the guidelines on page 39. Wear clean hosiery every day and avoid tight garters and elasticated tops which might restrict circulation.

Get professional help immediately if the skin on your feet changes colour or if blood or pus discharge from a toenail or break in the skin.

Professional treatment All diabetics should be under the care of a GP or a consultant at a hospital who may prescribe tablets to help the body's natural insulin to work efficiently. Many hospital diabetic clinics have an attending chiropodist to advise about treatment.

■ Dry skin

This is a common feature of getting older, when the skin is thin and papery in appearance, and frequently flaky due to the loss of moisture rather than oil. It may feel rough or be smooth and shiny.

Home remedies Daily use of an emollient cream after washing the feet will bring about an improvement, but because the effect of each application is temporary, repetition is essential. Suitable creams are Simple Ointment BP or a thick hand cream. You can also use a pumice stone or chiropody sponge before applying cream.

Professional treatment A GP or chiropodist should be able to confirm that there is no skin disease causing dryness.

E Exercises for feet, ankles and legs

☐ To strengthen thigh muscles, raise each leg in turn, keeping your knee straight and hold for a count of three. Then lower the leg slowly and repeat with the other one. Gradually increase the number of raises each day until you can do 20 with each leg. This exercise can be done when sitting or lying down.

☐ To keep ankles supple, point your toes and slowly rotate your foot around in a circle. Repeat the movement in the opposite direction, and exercise each foot 15 times in both directions. Circling is easier to do when sitting up straight with one leg crossed over the other; but you can also rotate your ankles when sitting or lying down and keeping the knees straight.

☐ To stretch the calf muscles in your legs, sit or lie down with your heels resting on a cushion and pull your toes up towards you, as hard as you can, without bending your knees. Hold for a count of three and relax. Repeat half a dozen times.

☐ To prevent a fall – before getting up out of bed or a chair – stretch your arms and legs a few times to get your system used to the idea of moving. As we get older our bodies cannot adjust to quick changes of position which is one of the reasons why older people sometimes fall as they get up after being still for a long time.

F Fissures

These are splits or cracks in the skin, usually occurring between or under the toes and on the heels. Wet fissures occur because the skin is too moist and loses its elasticity. Dry fissures occur where the skin loses its flexibility and splits under pressure – sometimes where hard skin becomes so thick that it cannot bend. Cracked or broken skin can become infected.

Home remedies Wet fissures should be treated twice each day with an astringent antiseptic. Once healing has started, daily swabbing of moist areas with surgical spirit will help to maintain skin tone.

For a dry fissure, apply an antiseptic cream or ointment, and cover with a dressing. Once it is healed, rub the skin gently with a pumice stone while washing, and massage with an emollient cream to keep it supple.

Professional treatment This is much as described above, but if infection has taken hold it may be necessary to treat with antibiotics. In the case of dry fissures, the chiropodist may use a scalpel to remove the dead hard skin from the edges before applying an antiseptic dressing. This may involve covering the whole heel with plaster for a few days. Treatment after healing is aimed at prevention, and will usually involve the regular removal of hard skin by the chiropodist.

■ Foot strain

This is probably most common in young and middle-aged people when the foot is painful, usually along the arch, and may feel cold and clammy as the skin perspires.

Home remedies Rest the foot on a cushion raised to hip height. Contrast foot baths may also help (as explained under Aching feet) so long as there are no circulation problems. Well-fitting leather shoes, preferably lace-ups, will give support to a strained foot. A figure of eight elastic bandage may also be useful, but check it is not too tight if the foot is swollen.

Professional treatment Your GP may prescribe an elastic stocking or crepe bandage for support and may refer you to the chiropodist, to diagnose which structures are strained and the cause. The foot may then be strapped to prevent excess movement and to rest it, without your having to stay off your feet completely. Made-to-measure insoles may also be prescribed.

■ Fractures and sprains

As bones tend to be more fragile in old age, if you stub your toes, drop something heavy on your foot, twist your ankle or fall, you may sprain a ligament or fracture a bone.

Home remedies Because it is difficult to tell the difference between a sprain and a fracture, you will have to go to the hospital emergency department for an x-ray. In order to avoid further injury while getting there, wrap a crepe bandage or headscarf around the foot and ankle in a figure of eight shape to keep it supported.

For a definite sprain, cold compresses help to keep down swelling. To rest the ankle or foot, keep it raised to hip level; for support, wrap it in a crepe bandage, which is not too tight. Once you can again put weight on the foot, be careful to wear a shoe that gives proper support.

Professional treatment Broken toes are usually strapped with sticking plaster, a broken joint or larger bone in the foot may need a plaster cast.

G Gangrene

This is probably the most feared condition which can occur in the feet, but it is uncommon except for people with diabetes or severe circulatory problems. If you suffer from either of these conditions, be aware of the danger and get professional advice about self-care and how to recognise a potential problem. The things to look out for are a toe or area of the foot which suddenly turns white, dark red or purple colour but does not return to its normal colour when the foot is raised above hip height.

Home remedies Avoid damaging your skin by exposing it to extreme temperatures of hot or cold. Report all sudden colour changes immediately to a GP or chiropodist.

Professional treatment This will vary according to circumstances, and may involve wearing a special dressing, taking antibiotics, bed rest or amputation.

■ Gout

This disease affects joints, tendons, the kidneys and ears and frequently attacks the big toe first. The onset of pain and swelling is usually sudden and is caused by a high level of uric acid in the blood – not as a result of overeating or drinking port and red wine. An attack may last four or five days; and repeated attacks may effect the movement of joints.

Home remedies, see professional treatment.

Professional treatment The GP will confirm that you are suffering from gout by testing blood and possibly taking an x-ray. Long-term medication may be prescribed, or just for acute episodes, and you may have to avoid certain foods or drinks.

A chiropodist may apply cold compresses for inflammation and advise about avoiding pressure and movement. After an attack, the chiropodist will stimulate movement of the toe by manipulation and exercises.

H Hammer toes

The most commonly affected toe is the second one where the joint closest to the foot becomes rigid, set almost at a right angle and frequently develops a corn on the top. Because the toe can no longer straighten out during walking, excessive pressure is put on the tip and under the joint on the ball of the foot. Both of these areas frequently develop severe corns, which may become ulcerated.

Home remedies There is no home treatment which can straighten a toe, so make sure that shoes are deep enough to remove pressure on the joint. It may be necessary to cut a slit in the slipper or shoe to relieve pressure (see page 68).

Professional treatment A chiropodist will treat various conditions that occur with hammer toes, such as corns. Insoles to cushion the ball of the foot and redistribute pressure and toe protectors may also help. Different devices suit different people, so if the first attempt fails, don't be dispirited.

As for curly toes, surgery is the only cure. The rigid joint is removed and the toe is straightened.

■ Hard skin or callous

A thickening of the outer layer of the skin is a protective response to excessive friction or pressure and can be quite normal unless it causes pain or discomfort.

Home remedies A pumice or abrasive stone or sponge will keep the skin smooth and, if used regularly, will keep the thickness down. Lotions for the removal of hard skin should be used with care. Coarse metal scrapers, razor blades and other cutting instruments should not be used, as a cut or break in the skin can lead to infection.

Professional treatment A chiropodist will advise about a change of footwear, protective padding or an orthosis to correct foot function. The chiropodist may also prescribe an ointment for home use or remove a callous with a scalpel or a chemical.

■ Heel pain

This can occur under the heel or at the back where shoes rub. For rubbed heels, see the guidelines about proper fitting on pages 60 to 63. Pain under the heel may be caused by the way you walk or by wearing shoes with soles that are too thin or with heels which are very hard. Pain also results from rheumatoid arthritis or sometimes from a heel spur, which is a small outgrowth of bone on the underside of the heel bone.

Home remedies If your shoes have very thin soles or an inflexible heel structure, try inserting a foam insole or a shock absorbing heel pad, provided the shoes are large enough for this extra padding. Reducing your weight will also put less strain on painful heels.

Professional treatment The GP may refer you for a blood test to determine a diagnosis of rheumatoid arthritis, or for an x-ray to see whether you have a spur. The chiropodist may recommended orthopaedic shoes or a specially made insole.

☐ Infections

These are caused by the activity of bacteria, viruses and fungi. The skin normally has bacteria and fungi on it along with minute mites – all of which help to keep it healthy – but when this balance is destroyed or the skin is broken, infection can occur.

Home remedies The wound should be washed with a mild liquid antiseptic and clean cotton wool – wash from the centre of the wound towards the edges, so that germs are moved outwards, using a fresh bit of cotton wool for each stroke. Dry the area in the same way and apply a sterile plaster, using an antiseptic cream or ointment. Unbroken blisters or burns do not need cream, merely a dry dressing for protection.

If there is a scab and you think that pus is forming under it, apply an antiseptic cream or ointment to help the pus break out. Change the dressing daily and inspect the wound. If it gets more painful, red or swollen, seek professional help. Diabetics should do this immediately if a wound shows no sign of improvement within 24 hours.

Professional treatment A chiropodist may first refer to the GP for an antibiotic prescription, after taking a swab for identification of the type of bacteria causing the infection. If antibiotics are prescribed, remember that the whole course must be taken. Otherwise some bacteria may survive and become resistant to that antibiotic. The GP may refer you to a district nurse or a chiropodist if the wound requires frequent dressing.

■ Insensitive feet

This condition often occurs with other illnesses such as a stroke, diabetes, poor circulation, or as the aftermath of polio. The feet are rarely completely without feeling, but may lose their sensitivity to heat, cold, pressure or pain. The ability to feel these things protects the body from scalds, frostbite and ulcers or pressure sores.

Insensitivity to pain may mean that cuts, broken blisters or bruises are not noticed and may become infected. The feeling of pins and needles is another symptom of insensitive feet and may result from a disease such as pernicious anaemia.

Home remedies At the first sign of loss of sensitivity, ask the GP or chiropodist to test your sense of feeling. If you cut or bruise yourself and healing does not occur within two or three days, get professional help immediately.

Pins and needles are usually relieved by massaging the feet and walking.

Professional treatment Damage to nerves is almost always permanent, and treatment by the GP or chiropodist will involve preventing further deterioration. Each cause of nerve damage will have its own special problems and treatment.

P Parkinson's disease

This affects the feet because it interferes with co-ordination and the sufferer tends to shuffle. The upper body often moves ahead of the feet, causing overbalancing and falls.

Home remedies To make walking as easy and safe as possible, footwear should be securely fastened, with the soles neither too slippery nor too rough.

Professional treatment A GP will prescribe tablets to replace the missing chemical which causes Parkinson's disease and may suggest physiotherapy and chiropody treatment.

■ Poor circulation

When this condition affects the feet and legs, they will be particularly sensitive to cold, cuts and knocks and will look a purplish blue colour after sitting or standing still.

Poor circulation is a complication of hardening of the arteries that carry blood to various parts of the body and frequently affects people with heart disease, diabetes or those who have nervous disorders or have suffered from a stroke. In middle age there may be a build up of fat on the inside of the arteries (atherosclerosis) or they may become hardened or less elastic (arteriosclerosis). In either case, the nerves, muscles and skin in the surrounding area becomes under-nourished.

Home remedies Follow the guidelines about clothing under Chilblains (page 15). Avoid knocking your feet or lower legs or injuring the skin, as the reduced blood flow means that the tissues are fragile and will take longer than usual to heal. Also avoid burning the skin with hot water bottles or by sitting too close to a fire.

Walking and exercising the feet will stimulate the blood flow, warm up your feet and reduce the purple/bluish colour.

Professional treatment If you have been prescribed medicine for one of the diseases mentioned above, follow all treatments carefully.

■ Psoriasis

This skin disorder affects the feet as well as the rest of the body. It is a non-infectious disease which appears as silvery, scaly patches, commonly on the knees and elbows. If the nails are affected, they become thickened and crumbly. Psoriasis often runs in families and can be made worse by stress.

Home remedies Keep the skin clean, and avoid any known causes such as stress. Nails can be cut in the normal way. Even though they are softer due to their crumbly texture, they can be difficult to keep smooth.

Professional treatment A GP or hospital doctor may prescribe ointments and creams which may have to be applied under polythene dressings. Ultra violet light treatment may also be used. Removal of the scales can cause minor bleeding, as the underlying skin is soft and fragile.

S Scalds

A scald is severe when the burned area is more than an inch square or if it goes deeper than the outer layer of skin.

Home remedies Immediately immerse the foot in a bucket or bowl of cold water, and keep it there for at least five minutes. If near a convenient tap, putting the foot under a gentle flow of cold water also cools the tissues and reduces the possibility of scarring. After the foot is cool, you can cut away or remove any clothing.

If the burned area is extensive, cover it with a light clean, non-fluffy cloth (eg pillow case, sheet) and go to the hospital emergency department for expert treatment.

If the burn is small, after cooling it, put on a clean dry dressing using non-adherent gauze, and keep a careful watch on the process of healing. Do not apply any lotions or creams, butter or bicarbonate of soda to a burn until you get professional advice.

Professional treatment The wound will be cleaned and dressed and pain killers may be given. An overnight stay in hospital may be necessary. The wound will need proper redressing at home to avoid infection.

■ Smelly feet

If a daily foot care routine does not prevent your feet from smelling, it is possible that you have the distressing condition called bromidrosis, caused by the action of certain bacteria on the sweat.

Home remedies After washing your feet each day, dry them carefully and swab them with surgical spirit, which tones the skin and makes it less soggy. A light dusting of talc will reduce friction on the skin, but too much will clog the pores. Contrast foot baths may also help, as explained under Aching feet.

A weekly footbath with potassium permanganate may help, but do be careful, as the solution will stain. It should be very pale pink to avoid staining the bowl and your skin brown.

Hosiery should be changed every day and should be of pure cotton or a wool mixture if possible.

Try to wear shoes made from leather or a poromeric synthetic. Leather shoes take about 24 hours to dry out after a normal day's wearing; synthetic ones take longer, so wear different shoes on successive days. Avoid wearing Wellingtons, or be sure to use washable liners or special insoles which contain charcoal to prevent smell. If possible, wear sandals which allow the air and sunshine to get to the feet. You may find sandals a good substitute for slippers; or go barefoot if it is safe for you to do so. There are also some footwear deodorant sprays, which may help.

Professional treatment A GP or chiropodist may suggest a stronger solution to rub on your feet and may have additional advice about footwear.

■ **Sprains,** *see Fractures.*

■ **Sweaty feet**

This condition is more common in young people, especially men, and may be caused by unsuitable footwear, bad working conditions or nerves.

Home remedies, see advice for Smelly feet.

Professional treatment, see Smelly feet.

■ **Swollen feet**

Swelling is common in hot weather and among people who spend a lot of time standing or sitting. The fluid which collects in the ankle is the watery part of blood, and the mechanism which returns the fluid to the blood stream becomes less efficient in old age, especially in someone with a heart condition. The calf muscles used in walking help to pump fluid back up the legs, but this pumping action does not occur when you are standing or sitting still. Swelling also occurs with a wound or injury.

Home remedies Sit with the feet higher than hip level so that gravity helps to drain away the fluid, as shown on page 6. Support stockings or socks may help if the swelling is only mild, and brisk walking in flattish shoes will increase the action of the calf muscles.

Professional treatment Your family doctor will diagnose whether there is an underlying disease and may recommend exercise or support hosiery. A chiropodist may suggest adjustable shoes or slippers to allow for swelling (see also page 6).

T Thrombosis

When clots form in the blood, they sometimes become stuck in a small blood vessel and block it. The condition is known as a thrombosis. A sudden blockage can be minor or have major effects, depending on where in the body it occurs. A stroke or heart attack may result from a thrombosis.

In the leg or foot the clot may block the blood supply to a tiny area or to a toe or the whole foot.

If there is an alternative route for the blood to circulate, then the damage is relatively minor; but if there is not, the situation is serious.

Home remedies Any sudden change of colour in the foot should be reported to your GP immediately. If you have had a previous thrombosis, be sure to take medicines as directed.

Professional treatment You may be prescribed tablets to slow down blood clotting. If a thrombosis occurs suddenly, you may be admitted to hospital for treatment.

■ Toenails

Bruised

If you drop anything heavy onto your foot, you may get bleeding under the nail which is very painful, as the tissues cannot swell because of the rigid nail. You may lose the nail after a time.

Home remedies Apply an ice pack to relieve the swelling and pain. Rest the foot up. If the skin is broken, follow the advice under Infections.

Professional treatment If you can get to a chiropodist or GP immediately, or within 12 hours, a small hole can be drilled in the nail to release the blood which gives almost instant relief. Some doctors will make a hole with a hot needle. There is little that can be done after 12 hours.

Care of nails

☐   Use special chiropodist's clippers designed for toenails, as these are much safer than scissors. Alternatively, use an emery board or diamond-faced file to keep nails at the correct length by regularly filing – moving along the length of the nail rather than across it.

☐   If you cannot reach your feet, cannot see well or have shaky hands, ask a friend or relative to help with cutting or filing. Be sure that there is enough light in the room, and put a towel under your feet to catch the fragments.

☐   When cutting start with the little toe first and check that the clipper blades will not cut into the flesh. For any accidental cuts, apply an antiseptic cream and cover with a gauze dressing. The next day check for any signs of infection and put on a fresh dressing, repeating this procedure daily. If the wound becomes infected, go to the chiropodist or GP immediately.

Damaged by disease

Nails may be infected by a fungus or show signs of disease from another body system. A nail infected by the same fungi involved in athlete's foot appears discoloured and crumbly. Part or all of one or more nails can be affected. Someone with heart disease may have nails with ridges across them.

Home remedies To prevent cross-infection, first cut and file non-infected nails. Nail clippers and files used on infected nails should be scalded with boiling water after use, and emery boards should be thrown away. A proprietary anti-fungal paint should also be used daily, but treatment will take 6 to 9 months at least.

Professional treatment A chiropodist or GP may recommend the treatments described under thickened nails. If the affected nail is removed, this will require follow-up treatment of the new nail with anti-fungal paint. Anti-fungal tablets may be prescribed by a doctor, but this is often less effective for toenails than finger nails.

Ingrown

A nail is ingrown if it has cut through the skin causing a wound which is weeping clear fluid, blood or pus. If the nail has a jagged edge (usually the side, not the free edge), the flesh of the toe may be pushed against the nail (by overcrowding inside a shoe or by stubbing the toe) and the nail will have cut through the skin (see also Involuted nails).

Home remedies To prevent infection, bathe the toe daily with boiled and cooled salt water or a mild antiseptic, and cover it with a clean (preferably sterile) dressing and gauze. To keep the ingrown nail from getting worse, wear a large enough slipper or shoe to prevent adjacent toes from pressing against the affected nail. A small wedge of cotton wool between the toes, away from the nail area, may help. A small pledget of cotton wool may be used to separate the nail and wound, but this must be changed daily and inserted with great care. No attempt should be made to cut the nail.

Do not persist with home treatment for more than three to four days unless the wound clears up.

Professional treatment The chiropodist may follow the procedure described above and may smoothe the nail edge, with specially designed clippers or a very tiny file. This treatment is usually effective in the early stages of an ingrown nail – hence the need to seek advice quickly.

If the nail has been ingrown for longer than five days, the surrounding flesh may be inflamed; and a local anaesthetic (given by injection) will be required so that the nail can be trimmed and the wound cleaned. In some cases, the chiropodist may also recommend a partial or total removal of the nail – done under local anaesthetic – and the destruction of the growth area with chemicals, cold or electrical therapy. Following this, the toe is dressed. The procedure takes about 20 minutes.

Surgeons have a variety of methods of dealing with ingrown nails – some may use the procedure described above, but many cut out the nail and part of the surrounding flesh, requiring admission to hospital.

Involuted

These are frequently mistaken for ingrown nails. If there is no trace of a wound in the flesh, you probably have involuted nails, where the U shaped curve of the nail is exaggerated and the side edges press down into the flesh especially when shoes are too shallow or short.

Home remedies Do not poke at the nail with a manicure instrument or orange stick, causing a wound which can become infected. Instead, gently scrub with a soft nail brush to clear any dead skin or dirt from the nail grooves, as this can cause considerable discomfort.

Don't cut your nails too short, as the corners may dig in even more. Cutting a 'V' in the free edge of the nail is of no use, and may catch in hosiery and pull the nail away.

Be very careful about footwear – if the shoe upper touches the nail, it will push the nail into the flesh and cause pain. This can happen if there is no fastening to restrain the foot, if shoes are not long enough or if the toe box is too shallow.

Professional treatment A chiropodist will clear the nail grooves and advise on footwear. He may apply a brace to the nail to pull it into a gentler curve. This is a long-term treatment and not a cure, but provides relief from pain.

The more permanent treatment is the removal of a section from either side of the nail to reduce the curve. A GP may refer you to a chiropodist or a surgeon for this to be done.

Thickened

As the nail grows from the area just under the skin immediately behind it, damage to this area – the nail matrix – results in distorted growth and thickness. If the nail rubs on the upper part of shoes or slippers, the friction may cause thickness and the nail may fall off, to be replaced by another damaged one. If anything heavy is dropped on the toe, the nail will also be shed and the one that replaces it may be distorted and thick. This condition is sometimes called a ram's horn nail.

Home remedies To cut a thick nail, you will need chiropodist's nail clippers but even with these you may find it too difficult. If so, file down the thickness, run the file along the length of the nail, not across it.

Professional treatment A chiropodist will cut the nail with clippers or perhaps with a scalpel, which should not be painful, as the nail has no nerves or blood vessels in it. A drill may also be used to reduce thickness – this rotates a small abrasive disc or cylinder at high speed. In some cases, the chiropodist may recommend removal of the nail and destruction of the growth area, to prevent a new one from growing. This procedure can be done under local anaesthetic.

U Ulcers

These open sores on the surface of the skin are raw and exude fluid which may be infected with viruses, bacteria or fungi. Ulcers vary in size, and are caused by friction, pressure, chemical or other burns, impaired circulation or loss of sensation.

Varicose or venous ulcers are common in older people and are associated with varicose veins.

Home remedies The area around the ulcer should be cleaned with a salt solution (boiled and cooled) or mild antiseptic, then gently dried and covered with a clean dressing. If the person with an ulcer is diabetic or has rheumatoid arthritis or poor circulation, professional treatment is essential.

Professional treatment A chiropodist may use a scalpel to remove surrounding hard skin (which prevents healing) and will then apply a dressing, with ointment or liquid on sterile gauze. Padding will also be applied to relieve pressure on the area. The chiropodist may take a swab from the ulcer to diagnose any infection and make a referral to the GP for antibiotics to be prescribed. A doctor, chiropodist and district nurse may all work together in treating severe ulcers.

If the cause of the ulcer is permanent, such as excessive pressure on the toes, the chiropodist will suggest the use of insoles or protective covers for the toes, once the ulcer has stopped discharging.

V Varicose veins

These are especially common among older women who have had children. They look blue or purple and have a knobbly surface, frequently ache and can bleed quite badly if they are broken by a fall or by a knock.

The swelling associated with varicose veins is caused by damage to the valves which help conduct the blood back towards the heart. Damaged valves leak blood which seeps back down the leg, putting extra pressure on the valve below. As successive valves fail, the knobbly appearance of the veins increases.

Home remedies Try to avoid standing still for long periods, but if you have to, wear support hosiery or elastic socks or stockings. They should be put on first thing in the morning, before the swellings have filled. When resting, sit with your feet above hip level so that gravity helps to return the blood to your body. If a vein bleeds as a result of a blow, lie down and prop up the leg and remove any tight clothing such as garters. Call the GP or an ambulance.

Professional treatment Varicose veins can be permanently cured by surgery, if you are reasonably fit. There are two main methods: injections and stripping. Both procedures involve wearing bandages for four to six weeks, and hospital admission is necessary for the stripping treatment.

Varicose eczema

This is associated with varicose veins and usually affects the lower third of the leg. The skin looks purply brown and scaly, or may be tight and shiny.

Home remedies Avoid injuring the fragile area. After washing, pat the skin dry and use a non-scented emollient cream to keep the area supple. Keep as active as possible to help circulation.

Professional treatment This will be similar to that for varicose veins, and the GP may prescribe special dressings or a healing cream.

Varicose or venous ulcers

These usually occur just above the ankle. They vary in size and can be difficult to heal because the skin is under-nourished due to the poor circulation. Once healed, the area will be delicate and liable to break open again.

Home remedies Prevention is the key word here. Try to avoid scratching, knocking or rubbing the affected area, especially if you also have eczema. If you develop an ulcer, see page 43.

Professional treatment A GP will treat any infection and may prescribe pressure bandaging or support hosiery. A chiropodist may remove dead skin scales.

W Warts or Verrucae

These are caused by a virus in the skin which forms a horny outgrowth, like a corn. One method of differentiating between the two conditions is to press down on the suspected wart, and then to pinch it. If pinching produces more pain than pressure, you probably have a wart.

Home remedies This involves the use of over-the-counter remedies which contain acid and may burn the surrounding skin and leave the wart intact. Perhaps the best home remedy to suggest is a general rule: if the wart doesn't hurt, isn't getting bigger, and you don't share a bathroom or go swimming, then leave it alone.

Professional treatment A GP may prescribe treatment as above or refer you to a chiropodist or dermatologist. The chiropodist will attempt to destroy the wart virus by using cold or electrical treatment, or with chemicals contained in lotions or ointments. Some of these methods require fewer visits than others, but may be more painful or be unsuitable for use on warts over joints. A dermatologist may use one of the above mentioned treatments or may cut out the wart, which can leave a scar and is probably best avoided on weight-bearing areas of the body like the foot.

A chiropodist or dermatologist may also use a laser to destroy the wart. This is a relatively new treatment and can burn the skin. If offered outside the NHS, you should make sure the person using a laser is properly trained.

■ Weak ankles

This means that the joints and muscles of the foot and legs are not working as well as they might, which leads to a tendency to 'go over' on the ankle and to problems with foot function. A professional examination may be needed for a diagnosis of the cause of the condition.

Home remedies These usually lie in exercising the ankles to strengthen them and in the choice of footwear. Flattish, lace-up shoes which enclose the foot are best, particularly a wedge heel or trainers, which have flared soles.

Professional treatment A GP or hospital specialist will explain if there is a particular reason for the weakness. Treatment provided by a chiropodist or physiotherapist may involve heat therapy, friction (deep massage of a ligament or tendon) ultra-sound and exercise.

■ Whitlow

This is an infected area of skin next to or under the nails and occurs when hands or feet have been immersed in water for a long time or the nails severely manicured.

Home remedies Keep the area clean and dry. A poultice of magnesium sulphate paste may help the whitlow to 'point' and burst, after which an antiseptic dressing must be applied. To prevent a whitlow from forming, wear rubber gloves for doing laundry and washing up; and don't poke at the edges of nails with sharp instruments.

Professional treatment A GP may prescribe antibiotics; and may lance the wound – something which should never be done at home. A chiropodist may suggest preventative measures and treatment similar to the home remedies outlined above.

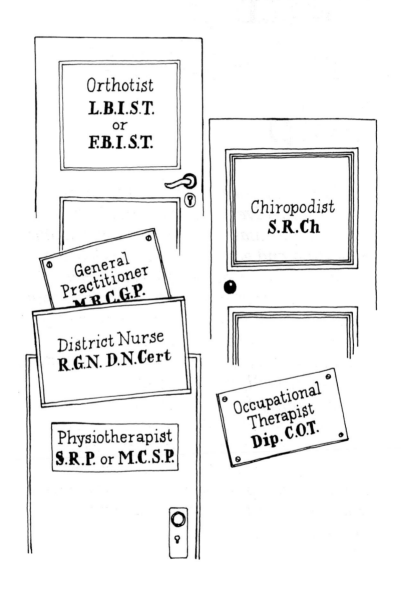

Getting professional help

Getting help from a specialist for a foot problem involves a partnership. You provide information about your particular condition and general health so that the professional can properly advise about treatment. Even though you may feel that you should not ask questions or take up time with information about yourself because there are so many other patients to be seen as well, you must take responsibility for your side of the partnership and explain your condition. Don't be put off when someone seems dismissive and says 'it's just your age'. Before going to the doctor or chiropodist, make a list of the things you want to discuss.

▤ Things to tell professionals

☐ Symptoms you have: when they happen, if pain comes and goes and when it is worst, what helps to ease it.

☐ Medicines you already take: your GP should know these, but if you are also under a hospital consultant, take the names and dosages with you (including any over-the-counter medicines as well) to all medical appointments. The chiropodist also needs this information, especially if you are diabetic or are taking anticoagulants or steroids which affect the skin and how it heals.

☐ Illnesses you may have: this is especially important if you have had jaundice or hepatitis, as there is a form of hepatitis which can can be passed on to other people through contact with blood, pus or other body fluid. If you are HIV positive (carry the AIDS virus) you should also explain this, to protect anyone helping you to look after your feet.

☐ Allergies you may have: remind the GP about these if he gives you a new prescription. A chiropodist will need to know if you are allergic to sticking plaster, particular ointments or dressings.

☐ What you want to know: advice about self-care for a particular problem, what to do in an emergency, how long the condition might last, what alternative treatment might be available, what causes the condition, if it is infectious, what leaflets are available to give further information.

☰ Professionals involved in foot care

■ Chiropodist

State registered chiropodists practice both within the National Health Service and privately and have the letters SRCh after their names. They are trained to treat and diagnose all foot disorders (including those requiring further hospital treatment) and to do this may use heat, cold, electrical or sound-wave therapy and prescribe the use of special insoles and padding. Their training also includes knowledge of diseases of the body which affect the feet.

To get treatment from an NHS chiropodist, ask at the local health authority or clinic or get a name from your GP's receptionist. Also check the state register at a reference library or look in the Yellow Pages. You do not usually need a doctor's letter or referral.

As there are only about 5600 state registered chiropodists in the UK, you may find waiting lists very long. You should get your name on the list and enquire whether there is an emergency clinic if your problem is urgent. Many health authorities have self-referral systems where an appointment is only given when requested by the patient, not as a matter of routine. If you are caring for a person whose memory is failing, be aware of this system to ensure that appointments are requested when they are needed. Many health authorities also run a nailcutting services, or the chiropodist may be able to arrange for a foot care assistant to cut toenails regularly.

Chiropodists who work in the private or voluntary sector also belong to professional organisations with their own qualifications, but many of these are not recognised for state registration. If you attend a foot care scheme run by a voluntary organisation or go to a private chiropodist, you should enquire about their training. State registered chiropodists who do private practice may also be on a list available at the local NHS chiropody service.

■ General practitioner

To get the name of a local GP, ring or write to the local Family Practitioner Committee; or ask at the library or post office for a list. Although a GP may not know as much about feet as a state registered chiropodist, she/he can treat infections and any underlying diseases which may be causing a foot problem and refer you for treatment to one of the other professionals listed in this section of the book.

■ District nurse

She is a state registered nurse (now called a registered general nurse) who may be attached to a GP's practice or work from a community nursing office. She is trained to give injections, change dressings and carry out other nursing skills requested by the GP, who must make an official request for her service. This may be done just prior to your discharge from hospital or for a particular illness.

■ Occupational therapist

The social services department is the place to contact for an OT to visit someone at home and arrange for the provision of aids and advise about adaptations for disabled people. Some OTs work in hospitals and you may be referred to her/him by the hospital doctor or your GP. Even though local authorities have a duty to provide an OT, there are often very long waiting lists for home visits and for aids to be provided.

In this situation, you could also get in touch with the Disabled Living Foundation at 380/384 Harrow Road, London W9 2HU for information about special aids and adaptations. You could also contact the Red Cross when special equipment is required, such as a wheelchair.

■ Physiotherapist

Like a chiropodist, a 'physio' may work within the NHS or privately. The letters to look for after a physiotherapist's name are SRP (state registered) or MCSP (Member of the Chartered Society of Physiotherapists). Those employed by the Health Service work from a hospital or in the community from a health centre.

Though trained to treat the whole body, a physiotherapist concentrates on disorders of the muscles, joints and ligaments. Frequently the aim of treatment is to build up strength which has been lost through injury, long periods of immobility or paralysis following a stroke. They can provide walking sticks, tripods and frames and advise on suitable wheelchairs. Many physios make and/or supply lightweight splints and insoles, special shoes for wear after surgery, and calipers.

To get treatment from an NHS physiotherapist, you will need a referral from a GP or a hospital doctor. To contact a private physio, consult the state register in your local library, or contact the Chartered Society of Physiotherapists. State recognised training is not required for a private physiotherapist, so be sure to enquire about qualifications.

■ Orthotist

An orthotist makes surgical corsets, cervical collars, foot supports such as insoles and surgical shoes. Most of them are contractors to the NHS, rather than employees, and thus may work for a particular manufacturer only. The orthotist will liaise with the hospital consultant, the physiotherapist or a chiropodist in providing insoles or in adapting shoes to a particular disability.

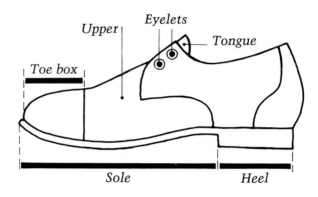

Toe box | Upper | Eyelets | Tongue

Sole | Heel

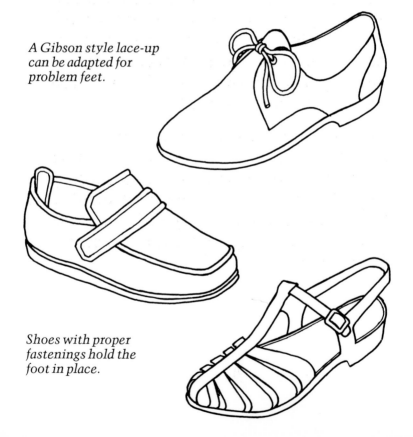

A Gibson style lace-up can be adapted for problem feet.

Shoes with proper fastenings hold the foot in place.

Footwear, adaptations and padding

This section of the book covers the factors to consider when choosing a new pair of shoes or slippers. The basic fitting points are covered with advice for people with special fitting problems or who may need shoe adaptations or padding.

As shown opposite, the selection of comfortable shoe styles for everyday wear is not limited; and there are ways to adapt shoes for people who suffer from swollen feet, need extra space for problem toes or who have difficulty in bending down to fasten shoes.

▤ Basic fitting points

Even though you think you know the correct size when buying a new pair of shoes, it is worth asking to have your feet measured for both length and width. When you try on a new pair of shoes, make sure you stand up and walk around in them. As soon as you stand up, your feet spread; and shoes that felt comfortable while you were sitting down could hurt when you walk.

To check that shoes fit properly, you could ask a friend or the shop assistant to help. Stand normally on one foot and go on tip toe on the other so that the other person can hold the back of that shoe and try to pull it off. Test both shoes. If either comes off easily, you have a fitting problem, which may be due to a narrow heel or unsuitable fastenings.

■ Length

Shoes should be approximately half an inch longer than your longest toe to allow the toes to move while you are walking. Even if your toes are very stiff, you'll still need this length as your foot rocks forward. The other important length measurement is from the heel to the ball of the foot, where the sole of the shoe flexes. If you have especially long toes, you'll need to have shoes with a long forepart.

■ Width

Shoes should be as wide as the widest part of your foot at the first joint of your big toe. There should be space for the toes to spread out when you walk. There is also the girth measurement to consider (around the foot) which is affected when feet swell or if you have a high instep.

For both of these problems a Gibson lace-up is most suitable – with extra-long laces – to help spread the pressure of the shoe evenly over the instep. For permanent swelling, choose a shoe with a soft upper to avoid cutting into swollen flesh. To make putting on easier – when toes are insensitive or paralysed – the opening can be extended down into the toe of the shoe and additional eyelets added for extended lacing.

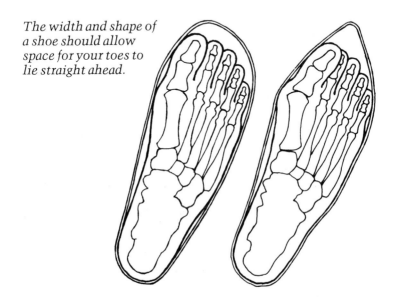

The width and shape of a shoe should allow space for your toes to lie straight ahead.

If you have a bunion, the width of your feet will increase. Choose a shoe with an upper which has no seams or stitching which runs across the area of the bunion, as the pressure from these features can cause blisters or small ulcers. If the uppers are made of leather and the shoe is only slightly tight, it can be stretched by a shoe repairer, chiropodist or physiotherapist to accommodate the bunion.

If you are unable to find a pair of shoes that can be stretched or adapted, there are 'semi-orthopaedic' shoes available from specialist shops which are made on a last with an extra-wide front.

Shoes should also be narrow enough in width to keep your feet from sliding forward when you walk. If you are wearing lace-ups, make sure that there is a ½" (1.2mm) gap between the quarters when you've tied the laces. If you have a low instep and the quarters meet, stick a small pad of adhesive felt to the underside of the tongue. This is invisible and can be done at home or fixed by a chiropodist.

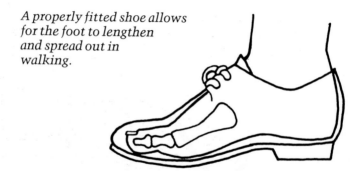

A properly fitted shoe allows for the foot to lengthen and spread out in walking.

The width of the heel of the shoe is also important and can cause rubbed heels. If your foot is particularly narrow at the heel, you can stick on heel grips or chiropodist's felt. The felt should be trimmed so that the thickness comes at the sides of the heels to hold them in place. If your shoes are not long enough or don't fasten properly, this can also cause rubbed heels.

■ Depth

This must be big enough to keep the toes and nails from being pressed on by the upper part of the shoe. If shoes are too short, or too narrow they will effectively be too shallow for comfort.

If you have buckled or hammer toes, it may be almost impossible to buy ordinary shoes with closed in fronts, and open toed sandals may be the only comfortable answer. This is obviously impractical for winter use, and you will have to look for men's or semi-orthopaedic shoes with extra depth or have a balloon patch inserted.

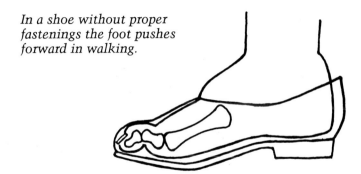

In a shoe without proper fastenings the foot pushes forward in walking.

Buckled or hammer toes will also be sensitive to any stitching on the toe box or a seam on the upper of the shoe, with a rough inside edge that may rub the toes. These toe deformities also cause pressure areas on the soles of the feet and may require padding or insoles and extra depth.

For shoes that are still too shallow for a problem like rheumatoid arthritis, a cross or hole can be cut in the upper part of the shoe – taking care that the edges of the hole do not rub the affected area.

■ Fastenings

These hold the shoe onto the foot and are most effective if they are situated over the instep. Laces can be pulled and tied to fit the foot exactly and are probably the best fastening. 'Touch and close' fastenings (two patches of velcro – one with hooks, one with loops) are also adjustable and are especially good for people with poor sight or arthritic fingers.

Straps with buckles are also effective fastenings – so long as the buckle is not attached with an elastic strap which cannot withstand the forward force of the foot in walking. It may be possible to attach velcro to the strap so that the buckle becomes purely decorative but the strap can be properly adjusted. A little loop can also be sewn on so that a dressing stick could be used to fasten and unfasten the straps.

Another alternative is a zip which can be inserted into the front of a shoe or a slipper or down the back seam. Either way, a tongue should be attached to the shoe to prevent the teeth of the zip from rubbing against hosiery and skin. Both the tongue and zip can be adapted for use by someone needing a dressing stick.

■ Heels

The maximum heel height for everyday wear is 1½ inches. As any heel height tends to push the body weight forward onto the ball of the foot, it is even more important to have an adequate fastening to keep the toes from being squashed into the toe box.

Despite the 1½ inch recommended maximum, it is best to gradually lower the heel height. If an older woman is used to wearing a higher heel, it may cause problems to change suddenly to flat shoes, affecting balance temporarily and causing pain in the calf muscles, which shorten when high heels are worn.

When considering heel height, the area which comes into contact with the ground is an essential factor – the larger the area, the more stable the foot will be. This is particularly important for someone with weak ankles or inrolling feet. A wedge heel provides more stability, as do many trainers and jogging shoes.

■ Soles

The slip property of a sole is an important factor to consider when choosing slippers and shoes. A sole which is too smooth may cause falls, but one with more resistance to slip may be equally dangerous in causing stumbling or tripping.

Polyurethane soles, now quite common, have advantages as well as some disadvantages. They have built-in cushioning to insulate the foot from the ground, are hard wearing, and are usually light in weight. Because they may be thicker than leather soles, they require some getting used to, to avoid tripping.

Leather soles can be repaired, but they may be thin or wear smooth and do not provide much insulation from the ground. They are not waterproof.

Whatever its slip properties and material, the shoe sole should be reasonably flexible – although there are a few foot conditions such as a stiff big toe which are helped by a more rigid sole.

■ More information

For more details about footwear and shops that cater for particular problems; send an SAE to:
Society of Shoe Fitters,
Farley Court, Farley Hill,
Reading, Berks RG7 1TT.

▤ Adaptations and padding

■ Adapting heels, soles and uppers

Heel sockets for calipers must be fitted
professionally, and can be added to commercially
made shoes. If the shoes cannot be adapted, the
orthotist may be able to fit a new heel for a
socket. Do note that you should ask the retailer
first whether he will change the shoes if the
orthotist says he cannot fit a socket.

Rocker soles are designed to help the foot roll
forward during walking, where it has lost some
flexibility at the ball of the foot or the ankle if
there is pain. An additional sole is added to the
fore part of the sole, thicker in the centre than at
the toe, so that the foot rocks forward on the sole.
It may be necessary to raise the heel as well to
maintain comfort. Sometimes just a rocker bar
may be added to the sole of the shoe under the ball
of the foot.

Shoe raises are inserted between the upper and
sole, are made of cork or a lighter polyurathane
foam, and covered in leather to match the upper.
Raises are added to the soles and heels of shoes to
even out the difference in length of the legs,
which can occur after a hip replacement operation.

Raises can be added to commercially produced
shoes, but you should check first before
purchasing the shoes. Many shops will allow you
to change unsuitable shoes so long as you haven't
worn them, but it is best to avoid this.

A balloon patch can be inserted in the upper of a
shoe to allow space for a bunion or for hammer
toes. A hole is cut at the appropriate place, and a
matched piece of leather is glued in, forming a
pocket to accommodate the swelling.

■ Lacing adaptations

Laces can be adapted for someone with the use of
only one hand or unable to bend down to their
feet, but a longer lace than the type usually
supplied with shoes will be required. To avoid
having to tie laces, there are also devices available
which can be threaded on, to grip them in place.

Shoes can also be laced with one hand by using a
dressing stick (a piece of dowel with a small
plastic coated cup hook on one end). Before
putting on the shoe, one end of the lace is knotted
and then threaded through the eyelets as shown
opposite. On the free end of the lace a piece of
velcro is attached below the loop.

When putting on the shoe, hook the dressing stick
through a hole punched in the top of the tongue to
stop the tongue being pushed back. The lace is
then tightened by pulling with the dressing stick

on the top loop, then on the next one down, and
so on, until the loop at the bottom of the lace is
tightened. A small piece of velcro must also be
attached to the side of the shoe, so that the free
end of the lace with its piece of velcro can be
pressed into place when the laces have been
tightened. To loosen the laces the process is
reversed.

Hooks can also be substituted for eyelets on lace-
up shoes, similar to the hooks on walking boots. A
knot is tied in one end of the lace which is
threaded from the bottom. A ring attached to the
other end of the lace can be secured on a small
stud attached near the top hook – after the lace
has been threaded around the hook, as shown.

Elastic lacing is a less satisfactory adaptation
because elastic loosens up with use and has to be
renewed. Elastic laces can be bought or made from
strong elastic. They should be inserted in the
usual way and tied, without stretching the elastic
to its full extent, with a knotted bow so that they
will not come untied.

■ Padding

Padding to provide support, redistribute pressure or cushion an area of the foot can be made of adhesive materials or be removable, as outlined below.

Adhesive padding should not be worn for too long, as keeping the skin covered does not do it any good, and the skin should be checked for allergic reactions. However, it may be essential to pad an area round an ulcer for long periods to assist healing, and the chiropodist will advise about material to use and the correct length of time to to keep it in place. Once the condition has stabilised, the chiropodist may suggest a removable type of material, as outlined below, which makes it easier to bathe the skin and keep it healthy.

☐ Strapping is used to hold dressings or thicker materials in place on the foot or to support or immobilise a painful joint. Strapping should be applied by a professional carer, as painful swelling can result if it is put on too tight.

Removable padding can be ready made or moulded from a model.

Straps hold padding in place.

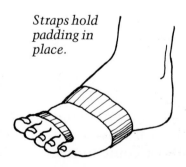

☐   Moleskin and fleecy web is used to reduce friction on the ball of the foot or on the toes.

☐   Foam padding in a variety of densities is applied to cushion parts of the foot where there is loss of natural fat or pressure from footwear. Soft, spongy foam needs to be replaced when it becomes flat, while the harder foam materials are more durable even though they may feel hard to wear.

☐   Felt is used to protect prominent bony areas such as hammer toes or to redistribute pressure away from painful areas. A cavity may be cut in the felt to contain ointment, or a dressing where there is an ulcer. A softer foam button may also be inserted in a felt pad to provide extra cushioning.

Removable padding   May be sufficiently thick to require your getting larger shoes to allow space for it. For example, a leather pad may be used to relieve pressure under the foot, to keep toes straight or to keep the shoe upper from rubbing the top of a toe. The ready-made insoles available to relieve a variety of problems range from simple foam cushions for the sole of the foot to thermal and anti-odour insoles.

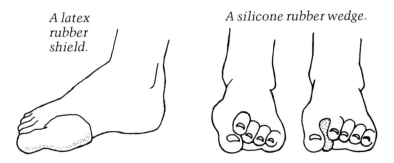

A latex rubber shield.

A silicone rubber wedge.

Many removable pads have to be specially made and require a model which is sent to a laboratory with instructions for the particular padding needed. However, some devices like the silicone rubber wedges to fit between the toes (as shown on page 71) are made directly on the foot.

Many chiropodists have facilities on their premises for making a model or the most common devices such as cushioning insoles to protect tender areas; functional insoles or orthotics to alter foot function in walking; latex rubber toe covers and bunion cushions.

■ Cost of adaptations and padding

There is no charge for these when they are prescribed by an NHS doctor, physiotherapist or chiropodist. However, if you go privately, you should ask about the cost *before* agreeing to have anything made to measure. The cost of appliances varies enormously.

■ More information

For a price list and order form about adaptations, and semi-orthopaedic shoes, send a large SAE to:
Disabled Living Foundation
384 Harrow Road, London W9 2HU

For more information about state registered chiropodists, treatment, and leaflets about care, send a large SAE to:
Society of Chiropodists
53 Welbeck Street, London W1M 7HE